Living Healthy

THE TIME IS NOW

AYAAN CARTHON

COPYRIGHT

Letter to My Hearts

One Team, One Passion, One Goal

First and foremost I want to dedicate this book to GOD, because without him there would be no me. I give all blessings to him, he have helped me come a long way through adversity. Through him, he gave me the strength, and knowledge I need to help others reach their goals. To my 7 children, and God daughter (Jordan, Dominique, Alexus, Jalen, Stacy, Tre, Destiny, and my baby Jayla) who have been through a lot with me over the years. Daddy loves you more than anything in this world; you will always be a part of my heart. To my nephew, my twin, I love you so much Nasir, your uncle is very proud of you, I love you twin.

To my mom a strong single parent, who has taught me as I got older, anything can be accomplished if you put your mind to it. Mom I would like to thank you for being that pillar I need to lean on. Thanks for being my rock, my mentor, my life. To my side kick my little sister, we have been through our ups and downs, but you have always stuck by my side. I want to thank you for everything you have done for me; I love you more than anything. I could not have asked for a better sister. To my baby sister Mikayla, even though I am not around often, I am always thinking about you. You are my heart, you are my life, and your big brother will always be there for you.

To my uncle, my father figure, when nobody else was there for me, you always showed me a better way. I thank you for being my best friend. I thank you for your guidance and support. Words cannot express our bond. It is something that cannot be broken, I love you to death. To my grandmother up in heaven I know you're looking down at your boy right now proud of the things that I am doing, I love you so much. Dad I know it took us a long time to finally get things straight, some days I wish I could sit and talk to you, I do miss you, and I love you rest in peace. To my auntie, I remember coming across the bridge, getting something to eat, and that love you had to give. Some days I wish I could talk to you, I love you.

Chapi, I must say through everything you have been a brother to me, and I will always love you. You mean more to me than blood could ever mean, through our Iraq days, and state side days, you are the true definition of a brother for life. Thank you for letting me have the honor of being the God Father to your children, that means a lot to me.

To my extended family Team Excluzive and Porter Enterprises, I love you all and thanks for supporting me through it all.

I had to save this person for last; there are no words that can express what runs through my heart for you. You have helped me through things other people could never have. You have been there as my biggest supporter. The faith and confidence you have showed me, means the world to me. There is no person that could ever take your place. Thanks for being everything I could ever ask for, thanks for being my best friend, my companion, my heart. Thanks for having the courage under fire to stick in there with me. Through the ups and downs, you have been there. I love you Princess K, PK/KP a direct reflection of each other, Te Amo Mi Amor Mi Princesa, my little me. There is a whole list of family, friends, and supporters I did not forget about you, I love you too, it's just too many to list.

I would like to thank those who support me through it all, and would like to thank everybody beforehand who purchased this book; you are making a difference to healthy living. Pass the book around to your friends, family, loved ones. Change someone's life today, do not wait until tomorrow. It can be too late then. Enjoy the book, and I hope you learned some positive things throughout the book, that can help you live healthier daily. Once again I appreciate your support. Follow me at dynastysports.co or my blog.dynastysports.co

love; Ayaan

Chapter One

The art of staying in shape is a lifestyle, not a hobby. Living healthy, there is no better time than the present. We always put things off that we can do today for tomorrow. Live life with a purpose, have faith and confidence in yourself, it starts with you. There are several key components that you must go through to get to your desired goals. As a Master Fitness Instructor I have seen a lot of people over the years reach their goals by listening to the different regimens, and programs that I have given to them. I have excelled on getting people to their goals. That is why I am sitting here putting it all down on paper for you to follow, and improve your lifestyle. Throughout this book I will talk to you about several different things, including why cardio is very important to our daily functions, why weight training is very important to us, and why having a healthier diet is the key to success.

First I will start by saying the very first important thing is to set a date when you are going to start your new lifestyle. Stick to your new program, remember the key component in all of this is discipline; you must have the discipline first. After you have maintained the discipline to move forward, you are ready for the dedication phase, and hard work. Recite these three things in your head, DISCIPLINE, HARD

WORK, and DEDICATION. These three things will get you far, when starting out with your new fitness lifestyle.

It might seem like you don't have enough time in your day for exercise, but you probably do, you just have to make it a priority in your life, remember it is a lifestyle. I have found out throughout my career as a Master Fitness Instructor, sometimes we have to set an appointment with ourselves to exercise. Pick out the times when you want to exercise, and schedule ahead. Keep your scheduled times with yourself, and do not let other engagements interfere with what you would like to accomplish. If you keep a calendar on your phone or computer, set alarms that will remind you of your workout time.

The best things I have found out that work, is by replacing something you really do not like to do. A lot of people have some unnecessary and not particularly enjoyable habit, such as watching TV, which could be replaced by exercising. Ask yourself how much time you spend on this habit, and whether or not you could exercise at the same time. Use it as a time to meet new people, or even catch up with friends, use exercise time to socialize. Stick to a routine, once you are in that routine it will start to come natural, after about 2-4 weeks you will find it less aggravating.

In life we must find something we like to do, find an activity you find most enjoyable. If you like exercising, you're more likely to stick with it. You do not have to just go to the gym to work out, you can work out outside also. You could try biking, inline skating, rowing, skateboarding, swimming, hockey, or any kind of sports; you could even dance in your bedroom with an iPod. Enjoyment is the key to sticking with it. I have found a good way to stay focused, and exercising, is by keeping a tab of your progress. A good thing to do is keep track of when you exercise and for how long. Make notes in your calendar, or keep an exercise journal. By doing this it will show you how hard you have worked, and how far you have come over the months. This will give you that sense of accomplishment.

One of the biggest things you want to do when you first start working out it set reasonable goals. Do not become one of those people who set the standards too high for themselves at first. A rigorous regimen right from the beginning, will not only discourage you, but also tends to make you want to quit. When starting to exercise you want to start at a reasonable pace and increase as soon as you stop feeling challenged. Try 30 minutes, three times a week and see how you feel. Avoid burnout. Working yourself too hard at first can lead to muscle strain and fatigue, and associating exercise with pain can make you more reluctant to work out next time.

As you go month to month remember to track your measurements. Instead of keeping track of your exercise success by how much weight you lose, try keeping a soft tape measure handy and measuring your waist and hip size. You might build muscle and gain weight, but you'll lose inches. Write down your measurements. As you start to trim up, seeing your progress can increase your confidence. Measure your neck, arms and ankles as well.

The key with weight loss, and trying to lose weight, you must learn to eat healthier, which we will talk about later in the book. The key to success with your new lifestyle is staying highly motivated! As you keep working out and building up your strength, your workouts will probably become easier. Don't allow yourself to get complacent, as soon as your current regimen feels easy, change it up and try something different. I am asked over and over how soon I will see results.

First, we must look at what do you think results are. Everybody results are different, and it dependent on your fitness goals. Some people exercise for weight loss, others are looking for weight gain, and most people are looking to tone their body. We need to look at some ways to determine our measurements, how your clothes fit, and measurement by tape, advancing to a more strenuous workout routine. Those are a few methods. There are several ways to measure your results and these methods will be dependent on your goals. I personally recommend you check your measurements, and weight on a monthly basis.

Sometimes in the beginning you might gain weight, do not be alarmed. Sometimes this happens in the beginning due to a fluctuation of carbohydrates, and water going to your muscle. You may also see a weight gain because fat is turning into muscle, during this period you will see inches. Sometimes you might have a medical condition so beware of certain issues that can arise.

You would like to consult with your doctor starting a new regimen, especially if you've had heart or lung related illness in the past. If you feel faint, dizzy, sick, or in pain while working out, take a break. If you start getting better soon, then just start once you feel better. If there is a serious pain or you're crying, you think something is broken, or it won't go away, stop and wait a few hours. If it's still not gone, call a doctor! People will tell you it is workout pain, but you know your body. If you are in pain that does not lessen for more than an hour, you should contact someone.

If you are in severe pain, contact someone immediately as it could be a sign of something seriously wrong. Consult your doctor if you are severely underweight, overweight, obese, or suffer from asthma before starting working out as you could hurt yourself. You should eat at least 30 to 45 minutes prior to working out.

Chapter Two

Cardio and or Cardiovascular exercise.
Cardio exercise works all of the large
muscle groups in your body. Cardio workout
can consist of walking, running, swimming,
dancing, cycling. By sticking to a regular
cardio regimen, it not only can help you lose
and maintain your weight, but it can also
improve your heart and cut your risk for
chronic diseases. First thing you want to do

before starting a cardio program is by asking your doctor if you are healthy enough to begin doing cardio. Cardio get your heart pumping and it also burn off those extra calories and fat. Combing cardio, weight training, and eating right, it can help you keep your weight under control. Doing cardio for just a half an hour of a day is enough to maintain your current weight. Your heart can benefit greatly from regular cardio exercise.

Cardio activities help to lower your blood pressure and prevent heart disease, and it can also improve the health of your vessels and vascular functions, allowing your blood to flow more efficiently throughout your body. If you have had a heart attack, beginning a regular exercise program can reduce your risk of having another, and it may even lower your risk of death by 20 percent to 25 percent, according to the American Heart Association.

Keeping excess fat from accumulating on your body can cut your risk of developing certain chronic diseases, and using cardio exercise to do this can provide even more benefits. Cardio helps fight off type 2 diabetes, and high cholesterol, and some forms of cancer. If you perform weight-bearing cardio such as jogging, it can lessen your chances of developing osteoporosis. Regular cardio activity also strengthens your immune system, making you less likely to catch viral illnesses and keeping your body healthier overall.

By adding cardio to your daily life, your stamina for other activities will increase, as well as your strength. This can help keep you active as you get older, and it can also improve your mental health. It is never too late to begin exercising, but you should always consult with your doctor before doing so. Tell them about any health conditions you have, as well those that are in your family history, and let them know if you smoke as well. They can help you determine how much cardio you can safely perform and give you tips on how to begin.

There are several methods to performing cardio exercise. Long, slow lower-intensity cardio exercise on treadmills, bikes, elliptical, and arc trainer is good for beginners or those who have been inactive. Research has proven that the benefits of cardio exercise (like sprint interval cardio) is superior to aerobic exercise for fitness and heart health. The progression of your cardio exercise should be low-intensity aerobics to moderate/high-intensity aerobics to high-intensity anaerobic exercise.

High intensity cardio and high intensity interval cardio training will give you faster body fat burn in less time. You only need to do 20 minutes per session, 3 times a week. High intensity cardio and high intensity interval cardio training will: 1) significantly boost your metabolism, during and after exercise, 2) give you less lean body mass loss, 3) give you a faster rate of body fat-to-energy conversion and 4) significantly increase your VO2 Max capacity. Circuit weight training (including bodyweight circuits) has dual benefits as a strength/cardio workout. If HIC or HIIT is too hard on your body, you might want to try a HIC, HIIT and moderate intensity combination during the week. Just get to know your body so you know when to back off.

The evidence is clear, if you want maximum body fat burn in the least amount of time, then HIC and HIIT is the way to go! Varying cardio exercise daily will burn maximum calories, and fat. It will give you muscle confusion, and keep your muscles working for you, instead of them reaching a peak.

Chapter Three

When starting a new health plan, you want to develop one that fits your needs. You're going to want to go to the food store and stock up on foods high in complex carbohydrates and lean protein. Good carbohydrates like whole wheat pasta provide your body with energy, while protein helps rebuild muscle, increasing muscle mass. Plan your meals around your workout schedule. Eat smaller meals before you work out and larger ones afterward. Eat meals high in carbohydrates an hour or two before you work out. The carbohydrates will provide you with extra energy during your workout. Eat a meal high in protein and carbohydrates ideally two hours after your workout, to help rebuild your muscles and provide you with extra energy.

Drink plenty of water all throughout your day. Water will keep you hydrated and is absolutely vital to keeping you healthy during your workout regimen. Drinking water is the best thing you can do for your body. If you do not do anything else please bring water to your workout sessions. Do not to drink excessive amounts of plain water after strenuous workouts, your body loses salts through sweat, and too much plain water can help to flush out whatever is left.

Sports drinks can be helpful for intense workouts, but consider the sugar content if your goal is to lose weight. Eat more fresh, nutrient-rich, healthy, low fat foods, rather than junk food. Junk food can range from burgers to cookies that you always bought. Adding a lot of vegetables and fruits to your diet will help you, they keep you feeling full for longer than processed food so you won't even feel the need to eat a lot during the day. Also, drinking broth, soup, will help you feel full. Go ahead and have that doughnut or slice of pizza, but before you do, drink eight glasses of water, and eat a bowl of raw veggies such as cucumbers, celery, carrots, and tomatoes. They will fill you up and you will have very little room to eat the junk food.

There are two things you eat and drink that contain no calories: water and fiber. The more of these you get into your diet, the better off you will be. For example, you can eat a pound of mixed salad with assorted raw veggies (carrots, red cabbage, celery, broccoli, onion, etc.) with a low or no-calorie salad dressing and only have eaten 100-150 calories.

This is because of the high water and fiber content of the salad and low calorie dressing. Also, eat lots of celery. It has only 8 calories; it takes more than 8 calories to digest it. So, you actually BURN calories by eating celery! It's not much, about 2 calories per 8 inch stalk. One thing you want to do is avoid sodas as much as possible. You can drink flavored water or unsweetened iced tea. Caffeine, when placed in a low-calorie beverage like black coffee or unsweetened tea, raises your metabolism and causes you to burn more calories. With that being said though too much caffeine has harmful health effects, so be reasonable in your consumption if you choose to have caffeine.

Doing this, and choosing what you put into your body on a daily basis, you can drop the pounds without going hungry. There are many foods out there that are proven to help you to lose weight, foods such as chili, green tea, berries and whole grain can do various things to help you to drop the pounds, by avoiding insulin spikes and keeping your metabolic rate going.

By adding broth based soups into your diet, it helps your body. They are relatively low in calories. By using good eating habits, it helps us with our diet daily. Always use utensils and sit at the table. This stops you from eating precariously. Eating with your hands will mean that you take in more food at one time. Don't forget to eat slowly and stop when you're full. A lot of us mistake thirst for hunger. By doing this we eat when it's not necessary. By keeping yourself well hydrated you'll feel hungry less throughout the day.

Throughout the day, spread your meals out, eat smaller portioned meals. If you eat 100-150 calories or so every two hours, your body stays in a higher-metabolism digesting mode. This allows you to burn more calories than eating just 3 meals a day. This is a simple method to success. Vegetables should be a major important part of your diet. Veggies are very important to weight loss. This is because vegetables are high in water and fiber and low in energy density.

Chapter Four

Weight training is an essential part of your routine. Start by lifting an appropriate amount of weight. Start with a weight you can lift comfortably 12 to 15 times. For most people, a single set of 12 repetitions with the proper weight can build strength just as efficiently as can three sets of the same exercise. As you get stronger, gradually increase the amount of weight. They key component for weight training is by using proper form. With weight training you must learn to do each exercise correctly. People must understand the better your form, the better your results. By having proper form, the less likely you are to hurt yourself. If you're unable to maintain good form, decrease the weight or the number of repetitions.

Remember that proper form matters even when you pick up and replace your weights on the weight racks. If you're not sure whether you're doing a particular exercise correctly, ask a personal trainer or other fitness specialist for help. Breathe correctly while doing exercise. You might be tempted to hold your breath while you're lifting weights. Do not do this; it is unsafe for you to do. Holding your breath can lead to dangerous increases in blood pressure. Instead, breathe out as you lift the weight and breathe in as you lower the weight. You must seek balance while lifting weights.

Work all of your major muscles, abdominals, legs, chest, back, shoulders and arms. Strengthen the opposing muscles in a balanced way, such as the front of the shoulder and the back of the shoulder.

During weight training you must rest in between, between every set you want to take a 30-45 second break. You must also avoid from exercising the same muscles two days in a row. You might work all of your major muscle groups at a single session two or three times a week, or plan daily sessions for specific muscle groups. Examples of this, on Monday work your arms and shoulders, on Tuesday work your legs, and so on.

When you're weight training, do not skip your warm up. If your muscles are cold they are more prone to injury than are warm muscles. Before you lift weights, warm up with five to 10 minutes of brisk walking or other aerobic activity. Do not rush through weight lifting. Move the weight in an unhurried, controlled fashion. Taking it slow helps you isolate the muscles you want to work and keeps you from relying on momentum to lift the weight. They to weight training do not overdo it. For most people, completing one set of exercises to the point of fatigue is typically enough. Additional sets may only eat up your time and contribute to overload injury. Sometimes it is good to work through the pain, if it is tolerable, if it is severe or moderate pain, you might want to stop, and seek medical attention. Try it again in a few days or try it with less weight. A shoe with good traction can keep you from slipping while you're lifting weights. Remember, the more you concentrate on proper weight training technique, the more you'll get from your weight training program.

Some key elements to weight training and important steps to follow. Always breathe out on the lift upwards. Exhale strongly and from the bottom of your stomach during the lift. A good strong exhale will help increase your weight lifting ability. Stretch your muscle before during and after each weight lifting routine. Stretch the muscle area that you intend to work out. If you are going to do arm curls, then stretch your arms out, to minimize the possibility of tearing your muscles. Move slowly during the lift and the return. Don't just rush the weight up and down, move slowly and use all your force during the lift. This will increase the muscle tone in your muscles. Move smoothly during the weight lifting routine. Bouncing or jerking the weight up increases the chance of tearing your muscles or injury to your muscles. Make the lift upwards and the return as smooth as possible. Follow through the range of motion during weight lifting. If you are performing arm curls, make sure you lift through the whole range of motion for your arms. If you stop half way up during the lift, your muscles are not getting the full effect and you end up cheating yourself. To build muscle you would want to go heavier and less reps, and if you are trying to tone, you would want to go lighter with more reps.

Chapter Five

A lot of people ask what causes muscle soreness. The exact causes are not known. It is believed that a breakdown of muscle fibers take place, while performing a strenuous physical activity. The muscle fibers can get some tiny microscopic tears, which in turn, can produce the soreness within a day or two after performing the particular activity. Such tearing can also be accompanied by inflammation, for which one can get muscle pain as well. The extent of tearing and the resulting soreness depend on a number of factors including, the type of exercise as well as how strenuous it is. Exercises involving eccentric muscle contractions, especially the ones that cause the muscle to contract quite forcefully, while it lengthens, have been observed to cause more muscle soreness in legs and other parts of the body. However, the same breakdown or tearing of the muscle fibers allows them to grow stronger and larger. But still, the soreness, stiffness, pain and the loss of strength associated with exercising can become quite annoying at times.

There are several ways that you can get rid of muscle soreness. Massaging the sore muscles gently and application of ice pack are two of the most simple and effective remedies for this problem. Even massaging the muscles shortly after working out and again, a few hours later can help in pain relief to a great extent. Application of ice pack and heat on the other hand, can ease the pain and inflammation of the muscles. In the meantime, it is very important take adequate rest, and by avoiding any grueling exercise or physical activity. But, simple and light exercises such as, walking and swimming can help to avoid muscle stiffness during this period. If the inflammation and pain is too severe, then one can take non-steroidal anti-inflammatory medications. However, for mild soreness and pain, it is better to wait for a few days, and let the soreness subside on its own.

Be sure to resume the workout program, only after the soreness goes away completely. For preventing muscle soreness, it is very important to practice warm up exercises prior to the workout session.

Gentle and slow stretching exercises performed before and after workouts can reduce the extent of damage to a great extent. However, some recent studies have shown that stretching exercises are not so effective to prevent muscle aches. Mild to moderate level of pain and muscle soreness after the workout session are quite normal, and go away on their own within a couple of days. But, if the pain, inflammation and the soreness seem to be severe in nature, and persist for a long time, then one should consult a physician to rule out the possibility of muscle sprain and other injuries. On the other hand, it is very important to go slow while exercising to reduce the extent of damage and minimize muscle soreness. This is the reason why, beginners should start a workout session with low intensity exercises, and then gradually go for the high intensity ones.

The most important thing to remember during strength training is to breathe regularly to establish a good rhythm. The biggest problem many have is not that they breathe incorrectly, but rather that they hold their breath. Rhythmic, paced breathing helps to prevent you from getting dizzy. Correct breathing technique helps to avoid problems with blood pressure rising too high during exercise. People are often unsure how to breathe during a particular exercise or lift. A general rule is to exhale under control while you are lifting the weight and inhale with control while lowering the weight or resistance. This sometimes puzzles people because the starting position of the exercise dictates the way you should breathe. Do not worry if you do the opposite, it is definitely better to breathe than to hold your breath during the whole lift. Holding your breath can skyrocket your blood pressure, make you dizzy and affect your performance and safety.

They key components to remember while breathing is for you to do not hold your breath. Breathing in reverse order is better than not breathing. Breathe out while actually lifting the resistance. Breathe in while lowering the resistance. Correct breathing does take some practice, but you will pick it up in no time.

Chapter Six

I will leave you with some important tips to remember. I hope you enjoyed this guide to a better and healthier life. If you cannot make it to the gym for a workout, take a walk during your lunch break. You can also do crunches and jumping jacks while watching TV, or pace while talking on the phone. In other words, take every opportunity to exercise. Your health is your most valuable asset. Politely refuse offers to drive you short distances with a car when you could walk instead. Don't worry if you're not seeing quick results. It normally takes about 8 weeks for results to really kick in visually. Remember, you can't do it all in one sitting. Regular effort, with enthusiasm, is the key! Consider alternative forms of exercise. Biking, indoor climbing, Yoga, Thai-chi, martial arts, etc., will all challenge your muscles in different ways, and provide some fun and variety.

Burn more calories playing than what you get from foods. Counting may help at first, but with regular exercises and 5-6 scheduled meals you will easily stay on track. Regular and moderate meals will keep your metabolism going. Go early to bed, and have plenty of rest on days you exercise. Muscles grow and repair themselves during the deep sleep. Play up-beat music to keep the pace and for motivation. Try not to exercise in the evening. If you exercise before going to bed, your metabolism is increased, endorphins are released and it will make it much more difficult to fall asleep naturally. If the only time you can exercise is in the evening, try to do it as early as possible before going to bed to allow your body to rest. Every day, make note of all the benefits you can perceive: increased energy, pride and so forth. Make it as long as you can and keep looking for new items.

Consult your doctor before starting any new workout regimen, especially if you've had heart or lung related illness in the past. If you feel faint, dizzy, sick, or in pain while working out, take a break. If you start getting better soon, then just start once you feel better. If there is a serious pain or you're crying, you think something is broken, or it won't go away, stop and wait a few hours. If it's still not gone, call a doctor. Consult your doctor if you are severely underweight, overweight, obese, or suffer from asthma before starting working out as you could hurt yourself.

Before I end this book, I will tell you that what you accomplished this far you should be proud of yourself. Now you have got to the part of staying in shape, eating better living healthier. Maintaining what you have accomplished is not always easy. Sometimes it is harder for others than you think. This is the part that you need to stay on top of, because as hard as it took you to get to this point, you can lose it faster than how long it took you to get here. By now you should be set in a schedule, and it should be a lifestyle for you. Remember living healthy and staying in shape is a lifestyle not a hobby.

You must stay focused at this point in your life. Have positive thoughts, as well as positive supporting friends around you. This is not the time to let up. Keep your mind thinking about the right things, the things that help you get this far. Now is not the time you can say I will go to the gym tomorrow. Now is not the time you can say I made it I can cheat, and eat what I want too. You are in a good state of mind at this point, Keep it there.

At this point you are making good decisions for yourself, about your job, your lifestyle, and your health. At this point of maintaining, continue to reduce the stress in your life. You have rewarded yourself with a new frame of thinking, better health, and a better lifestyle. Right now continue doing the things that you think is fun, the things that you have begun doing throughout this process. Remember your diet, exercise, and getting enough sleep is the key to continuing on the right track. Being sleepy reduces your concentration, increases mood swings. Do not allow yourself to fall backwards, after you have put the work in to go forward. Remember do not put off something you can do today for tomorrow.

Living Healthy: The Time is now, it begins now.

Once you change your lifestyle, stick to it. Getting in shape is as much of a mental test as it is physical. Establish ground rules, and stick to them. Keeping this entirely in mind, it is important to recognize that exercise isn't about setting a goal, measuring against it, achieving it and stopping. It is about making exercise a regular, sustainable and integral part of your life. I wish all of you the best of luck with your new lifestyle.

HARD WORK, DEDICATION, and DISCIPLINE

I would like to take this time and thank everyone who has supported me with this book. I hoped it helped you understand the meaning of living healthy and staying in shape. This is your life, and a way to live longer for ourselves, family, and friends. Once again thank you for your support.

Visit me on the web at
www.dynastysports.co

And blog at
www.dynastysports82.wordpress.com

For speaking engagements and seminars
email at:

Ayaan@dynastysports.co

Or

Maurice@teamexcluzive.com

Coming Soon

Living Healthy:

An Art to Succeed

About The Author

AYAAN (MAURICE) CARTHON IS THE CURRENT CHIEF EXECUTIVE OFFICER / PRESIDENT OF TEAM EXCLUZIVE POWERED BY EXCLUZIVE ENTERTAINMENT, DYNASTY SPORTS FORMERLY EXCLUZIVE TRAINING & HUSTLERS AMBITION CLOTHING LINE. AYAAN HAS A VARIETY OF EXPERTISE FROM PHYSICAL FITNESS TRAINING TO URBAN NIGHTLIFE EVENTS. EXPERIENCED AND WELL KNOWN MASTER FITNESS EXPERT, AS WELL AS EVENT PLANNER & COORDINATOR. AYAAN HAVE OVER 10 YEARS IN THE PHYSICAL FITNESS INDUSTRY, AND 10 PLUS YEAR S OF EXPERTISE IN EVENT PLANNING & COORDINATION IN THE ENTERTAINMENT INDUSTRY. AYAAN PRIDES HIMSELF ON EXCELLENCE.

AYAAN FOCUS TEAM EXCLUZIVE ON EXCELLENCE THROUGH GREAT